The Other AI

Finding your Superpower with Neuroscience

Jenni-Lee Williams

Cover image courtesy of Merlin Lightpainting

Edited by Brooke Goode

Design by Kelly Sinclair

A dedication

To all the incredible, strong, amazing, resilient and fabulous women I know: this book is for you – you know who you are, I love you and am eternally grateful to you all!

... and a couple of caveats

The neuroscience in this book is based on current research as at the time of writing. This research continues on and new data is coming to light all the time. I have, however, endeavoured to keep the information as up to date as possible.

I have tried very hard to give credit to all the wonderful authors and influencers that have helped shape this book. If, however, I have not given you due credit where it should be, please reach out to me.

Contents

Prologue   1

Part 1: Where did we go wrong?   6

A quick tour of the brain   10

Patterns and habits   19

Focus: The other AI   33

The social brain   40

Part 2: So how can we thrive?   44

Breathe   46

Eat   54

Move   60

Sleep   63

Part 3: Where to from here?   70

Resilience   74

Purpose   83

The final part . . .	87
Love, laugh, and live	88
Appendices	95
Appendix A: SOLAR © A framework for leading in uncertain times	96
Appendix B: BLAISE © The neuroscience of learning	100
Appendix C: All the brilliant books I recommend	106

We begin life on an inhalation and end life on an exhalation. Every breath in between is a gift: use them wisely.

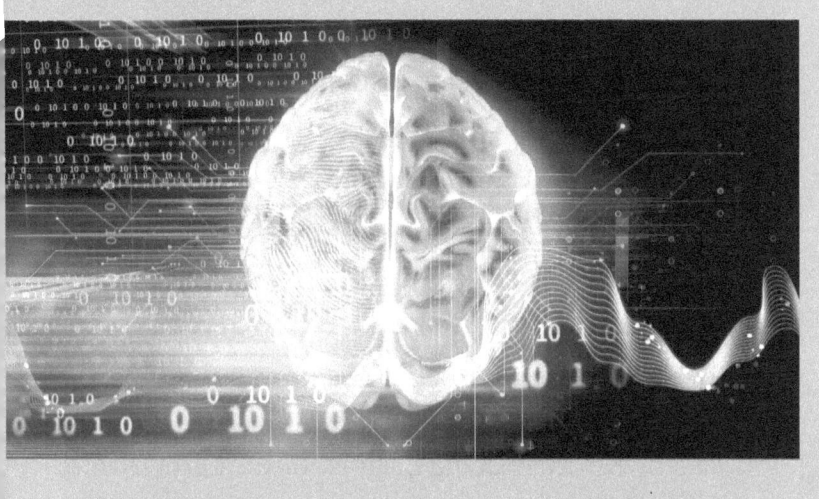

Prologue

Human beings are the only species on the planet who have managed to survive, and generally thrive, in almost every environment encountered. Our history is one of seeking out new experiences and places and inserting or asserting ourselves in and on them. Somewhere along the line, we forgot how to live our lives the way evolution intended.

Our brains evolved to move through our environment and experience new and novel things and learn and adapt as we go. They evolved to be social and to enjoy the company of others of the same, and different, species - as long as they weren't trying to eat us. Our brains evolved for us to survive.

This book is not a philosophical exercise, or a psychological one, rather, it is based on the readings and reflections of someone with a biology and education background and a passion for all things neuroscience. That said, these reflections are also based on many years of studying and researching neuroscience, which took me from Dr. Sarah McKay's Neuroscience Academy in Sydney, Australia to the NeuroLeadership Institute in New York, and on reading books by Norman Doidge, James Clear, Carol Dweck, Charles Duhigg, David Rock, Matthew Walker, Amy Edmondson, and so many more.

I have been fascinated for years by the quantum leaps and bounds that neuroscience has taken. As I immersed myself in the different aspects of the broad field, one of the things that started to become clear was that, while many authors went deep into the neuroscience research from their specific field of expertise, there were many practical implications for everyday life that could be drawn from each of them for people who did not want to wade through the extensive research and biological terminology.

One of the most revelational aspects of neuroscience is the concept of the plasticity of the brain. For a long time, this was a dirty word in all fields involved in the study of the brain, despite the fact that research decades before had proven it.

When I was at school studying biology, I was taught that if there was damage to the brain or neurons, there was no recovery for the damaged tissue or alternate routes for the functions that the damaged tissue performed. Now, we know that the brain is remarkably resilient and has an enormous capacity to reroute pathways to compensate for damage in specific areas.

In the times of COVID, I had to find different ways to exercise. Pre-COVID, I enjoyed aerial fitness, where I have a good laugh with a great group of humans with the side benefit of fitness and, as I am of that age, weight-bearing activity. My COVID-lockdown exercise routine, however, consisted of a round of boxing followed by a row on my machine, and, depending on my mood, a series of stomach crunches - sadly, no laughter involved.

I was doing the rowing component one day in September 2021, three months into the Greater Sydney lockdown, listening to my latest audio book and contemplating life, the universe, and everything neuroscience. As my mind wandered, I got to wondering when we forgot to breathe well, eat well, sleep well, and do pretty much everything essential for well-being well.

I have already developed several neuroscience frameworks based on my research: one to assist with leading in uncertain times, SOLAR © 2021; and one to design and deliver learning with the brain in mind, BLAISE © 2021. Both of these can be found in the appendices. I have also built neuroscience into all the leadership professional learning I design and deliver, as I believe a working knowledge of it is profoundly important for leaders.

In June 2021, during the brief window that we Sydneysiders were able to travel to Queensland, I was presenting on the neuroscience of learning and leading at a conference on the Gold Coast with a colleague. We had started with an ice- breaker activity along the lines of, 'If you could be a colour, what would it be and why?' As the participants introduced themselves and asked each other their question of choice, my co-presenter and I decided to participate. She turned to me and asked me the question, 'If you had a superpower, Jen, what would it be?' Upon thinking for a second or two, I responded: 'I do have a superpower, it's called my brain'.

The idea that you can literally change, not only the neural pathways, connections, and patterns and habits in your brain, but the size of different parts of your brain and the density of neural tissue, had been an epiphany for me.

So, I decided to write this book to explain the neuroscience and the practical implications of it to help people understand how their brain works and how to apply that to daily life.

I have written each section in brain-friendly doses so you can either read sequentially or dip into what interests you. I do, however, recommend reading Part 1 first to orient yourself with the brain and how it processes data and information.

This is not a self-help book. Rather, it is about how you can understand and apply what has been learned in the lab to discover your superpower, or what I call the other AI, Attentional Intelligence, so that you can live your life well and use each breath wisely.

Part 1: Where did we go wrong?

> 'Between stimulus and response lies a space. In that space lie our freedom and power to choose a response. In our response lies our growth and our happiness.'
>
> Victor Frankl

Human beings are protean. As a species, we are flexible, resilient, and able to shape ourselves to almost any situation we find ourselves in.

The story of the evolution of Homo sapiens is a remarkable one. We have explored and inhabited both hospitable and inhospitable environments, from the tops of mountains to the depths of the oceans and out into space.

As mankind moved via foot, raft, wheel, and wing, we took little bits of the past with us and managed to find ways to live in the present. We found companionship with humans and other species that we domesticated or used, in one way or another, for food and travel. We can actually track the movements of Homo sapiens across Africa, Asia, and Europe based on the genetics of the coat colour of the cats they domesticated and took with them. Or did they take us with them? You never know with cats.

As we moved across the oceans and land, we explored, stayed, or moved on and left our mark behind, for good or ill. We lived, laughed, loved, and ensured the perpetuation of the species. We fought battles, defended our hearth and home or stole others', invented and created new and wonderful - and sometimes terrible - things. Each generation believed in Gods, philosophised, learned, forgot and relearned (or not), and eventually died. But the species Homo sapiens lived on.

The brain size of Homo sapiens is larger than that of our predecessors and, we theorise (as soft tissue generally doesn't survive fossilisation), more differentiated. James Nestor, in his book Breath, argues that our bigger brain is at the expense of our breathing, as it came with smaller jaws and cavities necessary for freer breathing. Nevertheless, it evolved to be the brain that we possess today.

However, as Nestor mentions in his book, 'evolution doesn't necessarily mean progress, it just means change'. Some of that change has been to our detriment, psychologically and physiologically. The larger brain size came with a larger skull size, making human childbirth more difficult and more painful than for any other primate, according to the Smithsonian Institution's National Museum of Natural History. It also means, that despite the fact that the brain constitutes only 2% of the body weight, it requires 20% of the body's energy to run efficiently.

Maslow's hierarchy of needs has physiological and safety needs as the first two tiers. We now know that social needs are far more prominent than previously thought, and that the size of our neocortex, or cerebral cortex, evolved to encompass our social relationships or 'tribe' - roughly 100 people.

Somewhere in the journey, and I speak for myself here but suspect that quite a few of you will identify with me, we forgot the important things necessary for living life well. We focussed on work, career, acquisition, bigger and better, or as I call it, the 'stuff'. We fell into bad patterns and habits.

At the end of the day, you can't take the stuff with you. You also can't change your past, despite the attempts of many people to re-write history to make it more palatable. You can, however, live your present and influence your future, but only if you choose to.

Now I have enough Irish in me to understand that sometimes things just happen and that you can't always plan for, or account for, the unexpected. But should fate send the slings and arrows of outrageous fortune your way, you can choose how you respond and, in so doing, take control of the direction you go in next.

As Victor Frankl put it, 'Between stimulus and response lies a space. In that space lie our freedom and power to choose a response. In our response lies our growth and our happiness.' This is the neuroplasticity that is our superpower.

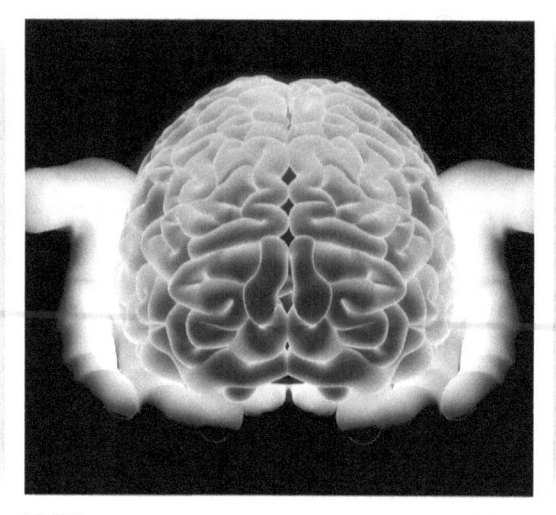

A quick tour of the brain

There have been many theories about the brain over the years that have since been debunked: the left and right brain theory, the triune brain theory, and the idea of a 'lizard' or reptilian brain, to name a few. I'm not going to delve into any of these here. I am coming purely from a brain organisation and orientation perspective.

If I were to put a brain in front of you, you would recognise the cerebral cortex (also known as the neocortex) or grey matter. The cerebral cortex is divided into four lobes, mirrored on the left and right hemispheres. The main lobe that we will be covering in this book is the frontal lobe, and specifically the prefrontal cortex, also known as the PFC.

The PFC sits behind your forehead and spans from temple to temple. It is where, amongst other functions, our working memory resides and is known as the 'Goldilocks' of the brain for two reasons. One reason is that it tires easily; of the 20% of the body's energy resources that the brain uses, the PFC takes the lion's share. It tires in around 20 minutes and tires at the same rate when you are making big, important decisions as it does when you are making small, trivial ones. In total, based on current research, there are around three to four hours a day when we can be in our PFC.

> When I was a little girl, we sometimes played a party game where an array of objects on a table were hidden under a cloth. The partygoers had a brief window of time when the cloth was lifted and they could gaze at the selection before the cloth was whipped back into place. You then had to write down as many items as you could remember and the one who got the most won the prize. Not as much fun as pass the parcel but more challenging. I loved the game. Clearly, even then, I was a neuroscience nerd; I just didn't know it.

The theory at the time was that we could hold up to seven items in our working memory at one time. This was eventually revised down to three to four items, and the latest research indicates that we probably can only be truly focussed on one item at a time.

The other reason that the PFC is known as Goldilocks is because conditions need to be 'just right' for it to function at its optimal level. This means that two hormones need to be present: cortisol and noradrenalin (or norepinephrine). Cortisol is also known as the stress hormone. Small amounts of stress for short periods of time help the brain to focus. Large amounts for prolonged periods of time are not good for you or your brain. More on that in Part 2.

Noradrenalin is, as its name implies, a hormone that puts you in an 'alert' state. In order for your brain to be functioning at its optimal level, both noradrenalin and cortisol need to be present in the right quantity. Too little and you don't have sufficient motivation to focus; too much and you struggle to focus. Mihaly Csikszentmihalyi describes this as a state of 'flow', somewhere between boredom and fear. Sadly, as I was writing this book, Mihaly passed away.

The other part of the brain that we need to orient ourselves with is what is known collectively as the limbic system. It sits under the cerebral cortex, roughly in the middle of your skull, behind your nose and between your ears and, like the cerebral cortex, has a left and right bilateral orientation.

Although there is some debate about what is included in this system, for the purposes of this book, I will identify the components of the limbic system and associated structures that are important to understanding how our brain operates.

The limbic system is often identified as the seat of our emotions. This is because several structures in the limbic system aid in the processing of, and emotional response to, external stimuli. One of these is the amygdala, made famous (or infamous) by Daniel Goleman and his 'amygdala hijack', or, as I like to call it, the open-my-mouth-and-stick-both-my-feet-in response.

The amygdala is responsible for our fight or flight, or in some cases freeze, response. I also read an article that mentioned the 'flock' response, which is to get to the middle of the herd and hope that the outliers get eaten before you do. From a business perspective, there is also the 'appease' response, particularly if there is a power imbalance present. However, this brings to mind Heywood Campbell Broun's quote: 'Appeasers believe that if you keep on throwing steaks to a tiger, the tiger will become a vegetarian.' It may work in the short term, but is not a long-term survival strategy.

Another component of the limbic system is the hippocampus, which makes connections with new experiences, stores our short-term memory, and processes our memories into long term. Because of its proximity to the amygdala, our strongest memories are often associated with emotions.

An area closely associated with our limbic system, the basal ganglia, is where our hardwiring exists, and this is where our patterns and habits reside. More on this in the *Patterns and Habits* section.

The overarching principal of the brain is survival. If the body doesn't survive, the brain doesn't survive and, from a Darwinian evolutionary perspective, the individual does not survive to pass on their genes. Consequently, the limbic brain is constantly scanning the environment to identify if something is a threat. This is happening at a subconscious level and comes online much faster than the prefrontal cortex and conscious thought (hence the foot-in-mouth issue).

These days, though, the threat is no longer the sabre-tooth in the bushes. Rather, it is people's facial expressions (including micro-expressions we are not consciously aware of), words, and actions, and the context we find ourselves in.

Living in Australia, I am well and truly used to snakes and spiders that can kill you, having encountered them many times (and written a book of children's poems about a large number of them - humorous ones, of course).

When I travelled to Ireland with my daughter in 2019, the cabbie that picked us up from the airport at Dublin was delightfully loquacious. He summed up Australia as the place where 'everything can kill you'. I don't think I had ever thought of it that way, but it's largely true.

We have a huge number of snakes roaming the bush (and our backyard . . . and front yard . . . and down by the creek . . . and under the house . . . and in the dressing room in the middle of the night, and . . . well, you get the picture and perhaps a better appreciation of where the poems came from). When bushwalking, you soon learn that if you see something out of the corner of your eye, it is smarter to assume a snake until you know it is a stick.

Fortunately for us, we don't even have to think about 'snake or stick?' as our limbic takes care of it. When the brain detects a threat, whether or not it really is, the amygdala will prepare us to survive, and we fall back on our patterns and habits.

Unfortunately for us, though, when our survival response is triggered in a work situation, our fallback patterns and habits may not do us any favours.

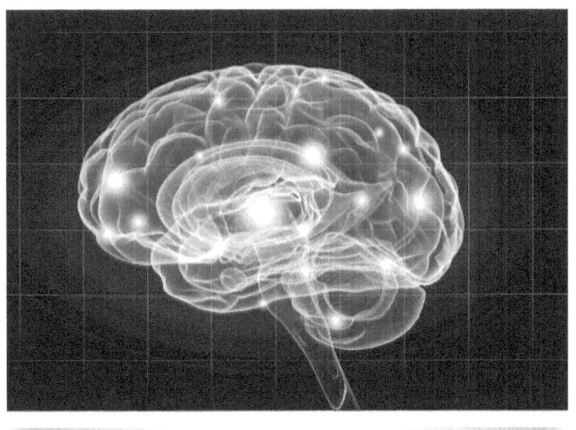

If you are the person who wakes at three in the morning worrying about things you can't change, you are simply strengthening your neural pathways to be really good at worrying. Now, why would you want to do that?

Patterns and habits

Mothers in their first trimester of pregnancy are generally exhausted. This is because they are building a human being. At the end of the first three months, a very small but recognisable human exists in the womb.

Even before we are born, our patterns and habits start to develop. In the first trimester, these patterns and habits are based on our genetics (nature). After that, they are formed by our experiences, the choices we make, the surroundings we grow up in, and the people we surround ourselves with (nurture). Even genetically identical twins will develop separate patterns and habits based on their choices and experiences.

Our five senses take in billions of bytes of data every minute. Some our brains pay attention to, and some we discard. Some make it into our focus and working memory, and some are eventually processed and stored in long term memory.

Have you ever heard a song or smelled something that takes you right back to a moment in time and a vivid memory and probably the emotions you experienced at the time? That's your hippocampus at work, making connections with your stored memories.

Because the PFC is so energy hungry, the brain has an ingenious strategy to deal with this. It moves information from the PFC to our hardwiring in the basal ganglia in the form of our patterns and habits.

These patterns and habits then drive our perception of the world. Consequently, I see the world through Jenni-Lee-coloured lenses. You see the world through your coloured lenses. These lenses are what make witness statements mostly unreliable, unless your witness happens to have a photographic (eidetic) memory. Even then, their patterns and habits will influence their perception of events.

The bad news is that once you have hardwired something, it is practically impossible to deconstruct it. The good news is neuroplasticity. We can overlay the old hardwiring with new patterns and habits. The more we focus on the new hardwiring, the stronger it becomes, until it is our go-to rather than the old hardwiring. You can also create completely new hardwiring; this is what learning is.

When I was undertaking Dr. Sarah McKay's Certificate in Applied Neuroscience and Brain Health (which I highly recommend if I have whetted your appetite and you want to delve deeper), Sarah challenged us to create new hardwiring. Yes, I could have done something highbrow and worthwhile like learn another language or a musical instrument. Instead, I chose to teach myself the cup song from the movie *Pitch Perfect*.

At the time, I was travelling into the city each day by bus. I didn't want to be the weird lady who sat at the back of the bus with a red plastic cup, singing to herself. Sarah had taught me that, to the brain, thinking about doing is the same as doing. So, I spent my time thinking about doing the cup song when I couldn't be doing the cup song.

Sure enough, around the 20-hour mark of both thinking about and actually singing the cup song, it became habit, and I had created a new neural pathway. Of course, every time I tell this story, people ask me to perform it, but no one needs to see or hear that.

Our patterns and habits come in four forms:

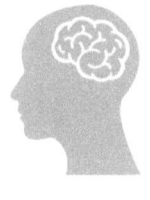

Simple and Routine

brushing your teeth, for example...

Although they do say that if you want to spark creativity, change the hand you use. You will come out of your limbic and into your PFC. NB: I absolutely do not recommend this for applying makeup.

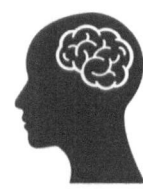

Simple and Novel

cutting a cake is simple...

Now you are at a children's birthday party and cake cutting time comes around. You have eight demanding seven-year-olds in front of you. If it has been a while, let me remind you, seven-year-olds can be ruthless about fairness. All of a sudden you have to recall your pi (to mix my food analogies) and work out how to cut the cake to have exactly even slices. A simple routine becomes novel again and bang, you are out of your limbic and into your PFC.

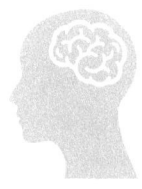

Complex and Routine

Ever driven from A to B and, when you arrive, you don't recall any aspect of the trip? It's as though you were on autopilot. This is a complex habit that has become routine. Of course, when you have to teach someone else how to drive, you have to pull it out of your limbic and into your working memory.

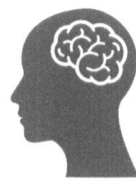

Complex and Novel

Now you are overseas, driving on the other side of the road to the one you are used to, and all the signs are in a language you didn't learn because you chose to learn the cup song instead. Now the complex, routine task has become novel again. When we were in Ireland, at least it was on the same side of the road we were used to. But in addition to contending with the ridiculously narrow laneways they call two-way roads and the crazy proliferation of large tractors using those same laneways, not to mention the abundant sheep, we had to contend with people coming around the corner on the wrong side of the road.

Once our patterns and habits are formed, they dictate our initial response when we feel threatened, as well as our go-to in times of stress. It's only when we realise that our patterns and habits are not necessarily serving us well that we may become motivated to pull them into the pre-frontal cortex and change them.

To change patterns and habits, you need the **three W's: the why, the will, and the way.**

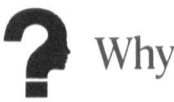 Why

Why do you want to change this habit?

What is it about it that isn't working for you?

Is it a routine you have fallen into that you worry about at three in the morning (more on that shortly)?

Do you come out of certain meetings with a certain person and kick yourself mentally for responding the same way every time?

Will

Even though, intellectually, you may know why you want to change, that's not enough to actually get you to change your patterns and habits. People who are told by a doctor that their patterns and habits are making them high risk for a heart attack know their why. It's only when they find the will or motivation, such as wanting to be alive to see their children grow up, that they will actually change them. When it comes to motivation, intrinsic motivation is far stronger and longer lasting than extrinsic motivation.

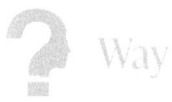

Way

Once you have your why and your will, you need your way: the knowledge, skills, and resources to enact the change. Remember, some of your best resources are the people in your life who care for you.

Habits are funny things though. You can't just wake up one day and decide to do things differently. Changing habits takes focus, hard work, and time. You also have to remember that old habits die hard and that you need to be kind to yourself if you revert to them, particularly when stressed. But as James Clear writes in his book *Atomic Habits*, 'Success is the product of daily habits, not once in a lifetime transformations.'

So how can we change our habits? Dr. Sarah McKay has a model called the four R's of habit formation: reminder, routine, reward, repeat. I have also seen the four D's model: discover, design, disrupt, direct.

Regardless of what model you like, once you have identified the habit that you want to change, here's a series of questions you can ask yourself to change the habit:

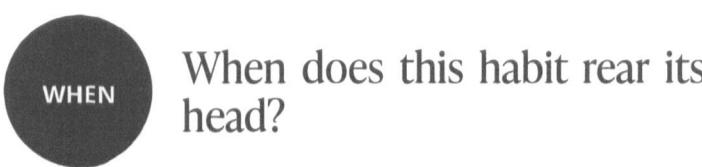

When does this habit rear its head?

What are the specific circumstances when this habit occurs?

Is it interactions with a certain person?

Is it triggered by a specific time or place?

On reflection, how do you feel when this habit occurs?

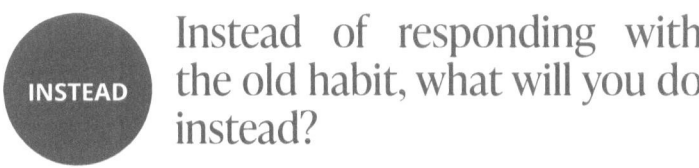 Instead of responding with the old habit, what will you do instead?

What will the new habit look like?

How will you feel when you respond with this new habit?

What won't you be doing?

How motivated are you to change this habit?

 How will you Stop yourself from responding the same old way?

Is there something symbolic that can remind you of the need to not respond the same way?

Can you take a deep breath or count to ten? Don't forget the power of the pause.

Do you have a critical friend that you trust who can give you the fish-eye when the circumstances arise?

 How will you focus your attention on the new habit when the circumstances arise again?

Can you and your critical friend establish a code word to remind you of the new habit?

Is there a visual cue you can use for the new habit?

What will you do if the new habit isn't working?

And just like that, I have come up with the WISH (When- Instead-Stop-How) model for habit change. I don't mean to be cute here but sometimes it's handy to have an acronym to remind you of what to do, particularly when you are stressed.

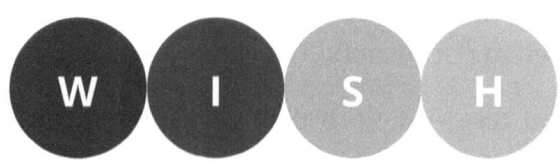

Once you have worked your way through these questions, I find this a useful sentence stem to fill out as a quick reminder:

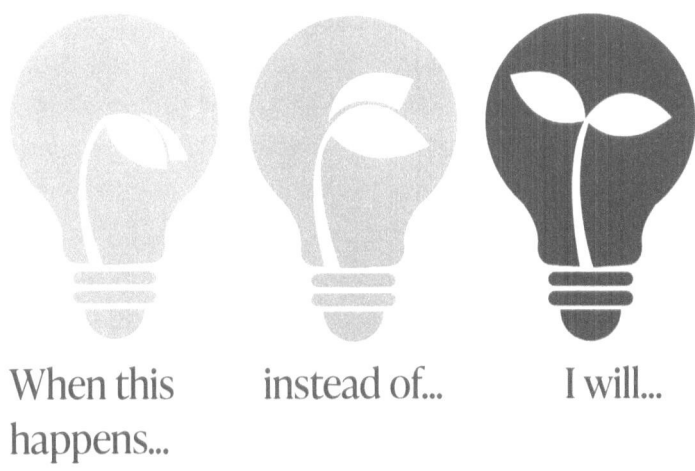

When this happens...   instead of...   I will...

It doesn't matter which model you use; just pick one that resonates for you and that you can remember, and practice, practice, practice.

There is also a quick-fix approach I have used to develop or change habits that is simple to deploy. It won't work for everything or everyone, but can help prod you in the right direction with minimal effort. I don't mean to trivialise habit change, but sometimes it starts with just one step and this is one I have experimented with and it has worked for me. You could say it's a bit of a JLW habit hack.

Say you want to drink more water or drink less wine or beer (I wanted to be alliterative here and say whisky but figured my husband would disown me). If more water is your goal, go to a $2 (or your equivalent) shop and buy multiple reusable water bottles: one for work, one for home, one for the bedside table, and one for the car (that you can drink out of without tipping the bottle up and taking your eye off the road). Keep them full of water. Some people say the water should be room temperature but eventually it will get there anyway, however it starts. Having them to hand means that you simply have to reach out and there it is, ready to drink.

If less wine or beer is the goal, but you associate a glass with the relaxation that comes at the end of the workday or social occasions, try 0% alcohol wine or beer – it has come a long way in the past few years. I am not talking about more serious dependency habits though for which you should seek professional help. However, if you substitute the alcoholic beverage with its non-alcoholic cousin, it can actually allow you to keep the habit without the health consequences. You'll sleep better too. If you want more tips about habits and how to change them, I recommend James Clear's *Atomic Habits*.

A final word if you are the person who wakes at three in the morning (it might be the alcohol!) worrying about things you can't change: you are simply strengthening your neural pathways to be really good at worrying. Now why would you want to do that?

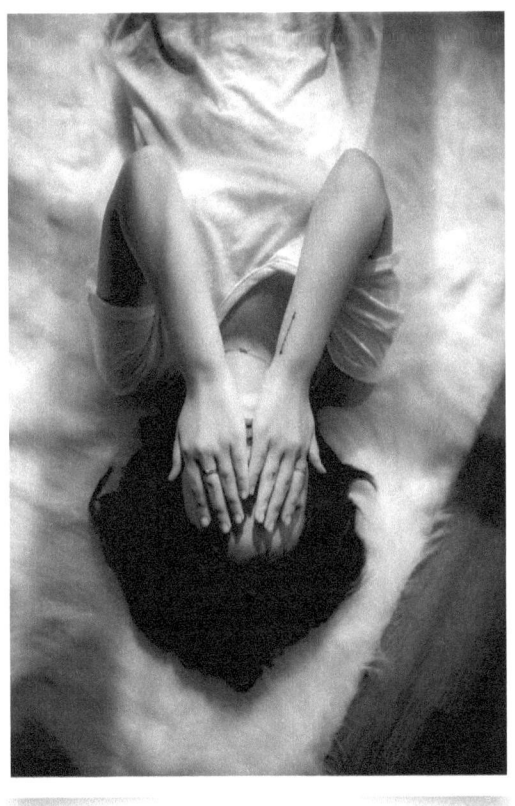

Photo by Anthony Tran on Unsplash

Short of the *Terminator* scenario, I believe what I call 'the other AI' - Attentional Intelligence - will beat artificial intelligence every time.

Focus: The other AI

The brain is both a connection and a prediction machine. It is constantly processing data, making connections with the sensory input it receives, and making predictions based on past experiences.

When you are fully in your PFC and have just the right amount of cortisol and noradrenalin, you are in the focus zone. If you think of your PFC as a torch, your focus zone is where you are shining the torch. If you are distracted during the 20 minutes you can be in the zone (as discussed earlier), it takes roughly 23 to 24 minutes to get back in the zone. I read an article recently on the epic business strategy fails of the past 40 years. Open plan offices were right up there at the top. Now you know why.

When I was a project manager at IBM in the 80s, I thought I was a brilliant multi-tasker. I know now that no one is. In fact, people who say they are great at multitasking are actually worse at it than people who don't claim to be good at it.

From a learning perspective, if you are within eyesight of someone else multi-tasking, you are distracted and won't be in your zone of focus either. Back to our torch light; every time you change your focus and shine your torch in a different direction, there is a switching cost. Effectively, instead of doing one task well, you do multiple tasks less well.

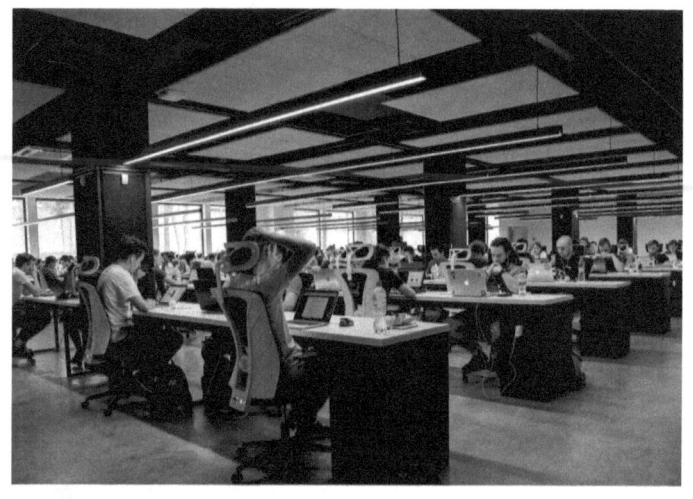

Photo by Alex Kotliarskyi on Unsplash

In his book *Indistractable*, Nir Eyal covers internal and external triggers that can distract you and what to do about them. Essentially, it is about being aware of what your personal distractors are in any given situation and dealing with them so that you can focus your torch. If you choose to procrastinate, then at least you are knowingly making the choice.

However, I did read an article once that argued a case for procrastination along the lines of 'it was the soldier that decided to stay in his tent and sharpen his spear or sword while the battle raged outside who survived to pass on his genes to the next generation'. Procrastinators of the world, you're welcome!

I call this focus the other AI: Attentional Intelligence. I believe it will beat artificial intelligence every time. We still do not understand the full processing power of our brains, never mind the ability for adaptation that is neuroplasticity. Then you add in the biology factor, fluid intelligence, reasoning, and non-binary decision making, and, short of the *Terminator* scenario, humans are infinitely more adaptive.

Our limbic system is responsible for what is known as our X-System, or refleXive system. Reflexes are those instinctive responses that happen without us consciously thinking about them, and are part of our survival mechanisms. They are similar (but not the same) as our reflex response to moving our hand away from a sharp or hot object. In the case of the X-System, it is your response to situations based on emotions, patterns, and habits. Daniel Kahneman, in his book *Thinking, Fast and Slow*, calls this System 1 thinking, or fast thinking.

The other processing system is the C-System, or refleCtive system. This system involves the prefrontal cortex or executive function, and is Kahneman's System 2 thinking, or slow thinking. But remember, using your PFC requires a lot of energy and takes effort.

Hebb's law states that 'neurons that fire together wire together'. In other words, the more you pay attention to or focus on something, the more your neurons will be firing together. This 'attention density' can shape your brain. Studies of London cabbies have shown that their hippocampus is larger while they are in the job and shrinks when they leave as they no longer need to hold all of the information to get from A to B to C in their long-term memory. Mind you, it takes them years of study to learn all the routes and there is a very high failure rate. Isn't that why GPS was invented?

We are what we focus on, and your thoughts really do count. What you think about and pay attention to can literally change your brain tissue. It can also help to regulate your emotions.

Regulating our emotions is an important part of living life well and there are significant consequences in failing to regulate them, both for us and for those around us.

However, if you think that being stoic and suppressing your emotions is the answer, think again. Suppression has an impact on memory - if you are supressing emotions, it makes your memory worse and means that they are not embedded in your long-term memory. These memories (or lack thereof) then impact our behaviour in the future. Suppressing emotions also has a nasty way of coming back to bite you when you least expect it, particularly when you are stressed.

But, I hear you ask, if suppression doesn't work, what can we do? I'm glad you asked! There are many strategies out there to help you deal with different life situations, and it really boils down to finding the ones that work for you.

If it is a thought that I cannot seem to get out of my head, I will sometimes write it down or, if I happen to be driving, I will count down from ten and tell myself (firmly) before I start, that by the time I reach zero, the thought will be out of my head.

If those aren't working for you and you have the time, take the troubling issue out into the light and examine it, look at it from all facets. In Appendix A you will find my SOLAR © framework, which takes you through a process to examine the emotions that go with the issue and then look at it to see what you can take away from it and reframe. Then put it on the shelf. Eventually, put it away all together.

Reframing, or re-appraisal, is a much stronger and better way of dealing with strong negative emotions.

It takes a village to
raise a child.

Unknown

The social brain

As I mentioned earlier, our brain size actually evolved to be consistent with the social interactions with our tribe - around 100 people. This is because, back in the day, being part of a tribe was vital for survival. These days, however, the need to be part of a tribe is far more subtle, but no less debilitating when we feel that we are on the periphery.

If you think in terms of evolution and biology, it is about survival of the species. From a sexual (as opposed to asexual) reproduction perspective, there are two strategies that species deploy: produce multiple offspring and provide no care with the expectation that some will make it to adulthood to reproduce, or produce fewer offspring and nurture them to aid in their survival. Part of the latter strategy is social. If your offspring can only survive with care and there is a possibility that you, as the parent, will not be around to provide it, social connections are vital. It takes a village to raise a child.

There are many mechanisms ensuring that these social connections form early so that, in most circumstances, the bonds will be there to assist survival. These mechanisms are both mechanical, such as breast-feeding, and chemical, involving more of those often-underestimated things called hormones, including what is sometimes called the 'love' hormone, oxytocin.

Longitudinal studies of the Romanian orphans that were part of the crisis in the 1990s have shown that, whilst they had food and shelter, the lack of warm and nurturing social interactions in their early years had implications from both a psychological and physiological perspective that reverberated through their lives.

Our brains have many unconscious biases, one of which is that we are more inclined to be friendly to and like people that we consider part of our tribe, or who are similar to us. We consider them part of our 'in group'.

HR professionals have picked up on this from the perspective of hiring. We are more likely to hire people who are like us than those who aren't. This bias is not always deliberate or conscious, although sometimes it absolutely is.

The focus on diversity and inclusion that is becoming increasingly important in business has its basis in neuroscience. It is only through understanding that we have inherent biases that we can seek to make them explicit and be conscious of them when making decisions. Someone recently described diversity as having a seat at the table and inclusion as having a voice at the table. My favourite quote in this area is by Shirley Chisholm: 'If they don't give you a seat at the table, bring a folding chair.'

There has been much research on 'in group' versus 'out group' and the impact on our behaviour towards those we consider in our group and those outside it. Being in the group can have profound rewards associated with it, on many levels. Equally, not being in the group can have devastating implications.

To the brain, social isolation is the same as physical pain. We know this from functional magnetic resonance imaging (fMRI - the colourful pictures of brain activity) studies showing that the same parts of the brain light up with loneliness as with physical pain.

The final thing I will mention about the social brain are mirror neurons. First observed in macaque monkeys, these neurons fire up when a particular motor action is performed by an individual, and also when that individual observes the same action in others.

It is still early (-ish) days from a research perspective, and so there is a reasonable amount of controversy around mirror neurons. There are also some grand claims, such as their being responsible for rapid cultural advancement in humans and our saving grace for communicating in the digital age. Watch this space.

Mirror neurons are also being hailed as one of the mechanisms for empathy. Empathy is a funny thing; it's a skill and therefore can be learned. I have read several articles based on a research study by the University of Michigan citing that today's college students are 40% less empathetic than college students back in the 1970s. They attribute this to digital devices with the rise of social media and the curated, and often augmented, life it can portray.

Remember I mentioned earlier that, to the brain, thinking about doing is the same as doing? Similarly, mirror neurons play a role in learning by imitation. We can learn to do an action such as hitting a golf ball by observing it and then imitating the action. Of course, how successful we actually are at it depends on a certain amount of talent and a heck of a lot of patience and practice.

People with good social connections are more resilient and generally live longer. It only takes one person to make a difference. You can be that one person in other people's lives and be greatly rewarded in yours in the process.

Part 2: So how can we thrive?

...do (mostly) everything in moderation.

For the remainder of this book, I am going to take you on a journey of various aspects of living life well. It comes with a caveat though; if you want to change your patterns and habits, you need to find what works for you, and your why, will, and way. It also comes with the overarching advice to do (mostly) everything in moderation.

Breathe

I always used to think it was amusing when people would give the advice of 'just breathe'. Now I understand the power behind those two little words and that we often forget to do just that. There's a reason why breathing patterns are taught to pregnant women to help with the pain of child-birth.

Over the years, I have struggled to find my own form of mindfulness. I have journaled with some success, tried various techniques such as imagining my thoughts as leaves that I scatter on the river flowing through my mind, or floating on an ocean of light, not to mention listening to all the sounds around me to hear beyond my own beating heart and growling stomach.

I am not trying to trivialise these techniques, but they simply did not work for me. My busy little brain would be jumping around from point to point, thinking about all the things that needed to be done and going off on seemingly random tangents that only made sense to me and did nothing to calm my mind. I felt a little like the dog in the movie *Up* with his 'squirrel'. If you haven't seen this movie, I recommend it but bring a box of tissues.

Before I knew it, time had passed, and I felt no better than when I started trying to practice mindfulness in the first place. More often than not, I would be frustrated because all the things on my to-do list had popped into my head and here I was 'wasting' time!

Here's where a little knowledge can be a dangerous thing. I know, from a neuroscience perspective, that mindfulness techniques are a really powerful way to help focus your brain and your AI, harnessing your superpower. They are also extremely helpful in lowering cortisol levels, and have been shown to have positive impacts on overall health and well-being.

Over the years, I have found a few that did make a difference and that I would recommend. But I come back to the point I made above; you have to find what works for you. The one thing they have in common is they all involve breathing as a component.

I have found the following quick technique does work and can pretty much be done anywhere, taking as little or as long as you like.

Start by getting comfortable in a chair or on the ground. I like to close my eyes so I block out visual stimulus. Start with a body scan either from the top of your head down to the toes or vice versa. As you move down or up, clench the muscles in that area and then actively release them. This will allow you to identify tensions and let them go.

We all carry tensions in different parts of the body and sometimes we don't even know we are carrying them. I tend to carry it in my neck and jaw so I usually roll my neck and shoulders and consciously unclench my jaw.

Once I have done my scan, I like to take three deep breaths in through the nose and out through the mouth. Then, depending on what I need to achieve, I will undertake different breathing techniques. Andrew Huberman *(The Huberman Lab Podcast)* advocates for the physiological sigh: breathe in deeply through your nose and then, when you think you have breathed in as much as you can, take one more short, sharp (noisy) breath in through the nose. Then let your breath out (again, noisily) through your mouth. This noisy out-breath is also called dragon breathing.

There are three main categories that breathing techniques fit into: **water, whisky, and coffee** breathing. Water breathing can be used any time of the night or day, and essentially slows down your breaths per minute. Whisky breathing should only be used when you are deliberately trying to relax or go to sleep, and coffee breathing should be done sparingly to make you more alert.

Water - Sit comfortably, inhale through the nose and exhale through the nose to a count of four each time. This regulates your breathing to four to six breaths per minute, which balances your nervous system.

Whisky - This breathing is usually a shorter in-breath than out-breath, such as inhaling to four and breathing out to eight. When you breathe in, you engage your sympathetic nervous system. This is your fight-or-flight system. When you breathe out, your parasympathetic system is engaged, which has a calming effect. This is why most forms of relaxation breathing focus on a longer exhale and slowing the breath in general. This slows your heart rate, reduces blood pressure, and helps you to relax and go to sleep.

Coffee - Focus on the out-breath only. Don't inhale, just exhale sharply though your nose to a count of 20. It's almost like a sneeze. You can feel the work happening in the abdomen. It can make you agitated if you use it too frequently. Do three rounds of 20 in the morning and again before exercise, or at 2:17 p.m. - apparently the time in the afternoon that we hit an energy low - rather than going for a sugar hit.

If I need to reduce anxiety and the cortisol levels in my brain, my go-to is what is called box breathing, which is a type of whisky breathing. I was drawn to it initially because I read an article that said U.S. Navy SEALS used the technique and I thought that was cool. I also liked it because you can pretty much do it anywhere, and no one knows you are doing it.

Remember the weird lady at the back of the bus with the cup? I also didn't want to be the weird lady at the back of the bus with her eyes closed doing strange breathing techniques. I have found it useful, too, in meetings where I just needed to take a moment and pause before I resorted to patterns and habits that would have negative repercussions for my career (my foot-in-mouth response).

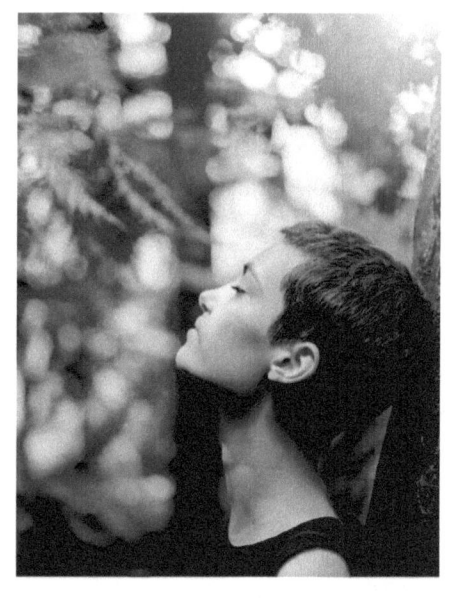

Photo by Motoki Tonn on Unsplash

Another reason I like box breathing is purely pragmatic; I am so busy counting my breaths and remembering what comes next that there is no room for other random thoughts to flit through my brain. So, if you are comfortable and would like to give it a go, follow me.

It's called box or square breathing because you can imagine a box and do the count at a pace that works for you. So, breathe out to begin, then:

Breathe in, two, three, four…

Hold, two, three, four…

Breathe out, two, three, four…

Hold, two, three, four…

Repeat this set of instructions for at least two minutes, preferably five. Box breathing can be helpful to get to sleep, or get back to sleep if you've done the 3 a.m. wake-up thing.

Unless you are doing deliberate water breathing, it's really important to breathe in through the nose and out through the mouth. Despite the annoying aspects of those nose hairs, they are there for a reason. They are part of the body's first line of defence against invasion and help to filter particulates out of the air.

If you are interested in discovering more about breathing and the effects of slow breathing and mouth breathing, I recommend James Nestor's *Breath*.

'Eat food, mostly plants,
not too much.'

Michael Pollen

Eat

Did you know that when doctors question you regarding your eating and drinking habits, they don't believe your answers and add a multiplying factor? Apparently, this is why diet studies are so difficult, as we tend to fabricate our responses in a desire to come across as more moderate than we actually are.

Blue Zones (so named because a blue marker was used to identify them - just as well there are no puce markers) are places in the world where the life expectancy is higher than elsewhere, and that have more centenarians in their population than average. They are places such as Sardinia, Okinawa, and Costa Rica, to name a few.

Research on these areas indicates that variations on the Mediterranean diet are probably the best for overall health and well-being. Hearteningly, at least for me, these variations do include such things as coffee and wine.

However, these zones also have other aspects that factor in: people who live in them are more active, do not overeat, and modulate how much they eat, what they eat, and when they eat. They also have strong social connections. And you can't discount genetics and the patterns and habits that they developed.

Evolution has also meant that our digestive tracts have changed and we are left with 'hangovers', or vestigial structures, that can sometimes cause us problems. Not everyone has four wisdom teeth: some have three, two, one, or none. This is because we no longer need large surfaces to grind up the tough food we once ate. That's not to say, though, that most of us shouldn't chew our food more, as a mechanical way to break down some of the tougher food that we should be eating as part of the Mediterranean diet. Chewing also allows you to slow down your eating so that your brain has a chance to catch up when your gut signals 'I'm full'.

Our appendix, which can sometimes cause us grief, is also a leftover from our plant-eating days. Cellulose, found in plants, is a very tough molecule to break down. Cows deal with it with four stomachs and chewing their cud; birds deal with it by having grit in their crops for mechanical breakdown, and termites have special microorganisms in their gut to aid in the breakdown of our houses (just another one of the joyful critters we have at our place).

Koalas have an interesting and rare solution to the tough, waxy, essentially toxic eucalyptus leaves that they love so much. Joeys are not born with the microorganisms in their gut necessary to digest the leaves and extract the nutrients. So, they are fed faecal matter as they are being weaned so they can gain the necessary gut flora. Glad you're not a koala?

You may have heard of the gut brain or gut mind connection. Most of you will know of your central nervous system (CNS) and peripheral nervous system (PNS). What you may not know is that you also have an enteric nervous system (ENS). This system of neurons lines your gut. Whilst it does not control our conscious thoughts, it communicates with our brain and can have a significant impact on our digestion, mood, health, and even our subconscious thoughts.

Those 'butterflies' in your stomach are a result of this communication, and indicate heightened anxiety. Similarly, it may sometimes be difficult to focus your prefrontal cortex when you are hungry, as your stomach is redirecting your focus and attention.

Research into the CNS/ENS interaction is continuing with investigations into such conditions as irritable bowel syndrome (IBS) and its connections to depression. But which is the chicken and which is the egg? Do people with IBS suffer from increased anxiety and depression or do people with depression and anxiety suffer from IBS?

To better understand your body, think of it as a closed system. Everything in the system is connected to everything else and there is a Chaos Theory kind of butterfly effect that occurs; something happening in one part of the system can have a profound effect elsewhere in the system. Things entering the system that should (food and drink) or should not (pathogens such as bacteria and viruses) be there can also have a profound effect.

A classic example of this is a disease that Australia has the distinction of having the highest rate of: mammalian meat allergy (MMA). This is a disease that comes about when you have had too many tick bites and is near, and not so dear, to my heart, as I have it.

As the tick latches on, it regurgitates blood from other animals it has been sucking on, such as bandicoots. As it does this, it introduces a sugar called alpha galactose into our blood stream, which causes MMA in some people. End result: you can no longer eat mammals and need to keep to things that fly, swim, or crawl. On a side-note, you can eat humans so you don't want to be stranded on a desert island with me.

I am going to borrow an old programming saying that is 'garbage in, garbage out' or, put simply, you are what you eat. Your digestive system, starting with your teeth (mechanical) and saliva (chemical), breaks down the food and drink you eat into basic sugars (carbohydrates), proteins, and fats. These are used for various things in the body, including making more of you. The more processed the food you eat, generally, the less nutrients you will be able to extract and the less your system is able to do the job it was designed to do.

The next time you are cursing fats, remember that they are usually what adds the flavour to food, are necessary for cushioning your internal organs, and are an essential component for your immune system. Not only that, but your brain is also made of approximately 60% fat. What's known as the white matter in our brains is the myelin sheath, which is comprised of fat. Myelin coats the neurons and its deterioration is the culprit in diseases such as multiple sclerosis (sclerosis being the hardening of the myelin sheath so that the electrochemical signal does not move the way or at the rate that it should).

I cannot finish this section without talking about water. Our bodies are made up of around 60% water. It is the universal solvent and, once we have broken down what we eat, quite a few of the constituents travel around the body to where they are needed dissolved in water.

Our blood is also comprised of around 90% water, and water is an essential component in many of the biochemical processes that make up our metabolism. I heard recently a rule of thumb: two litres before 2pm.

So, to end where I began, eat (mostly) everything in moderation. Or, as Michael Pollan says, 'Eat food, mostly plants, not too much' and drink, drink, drink - water of course!

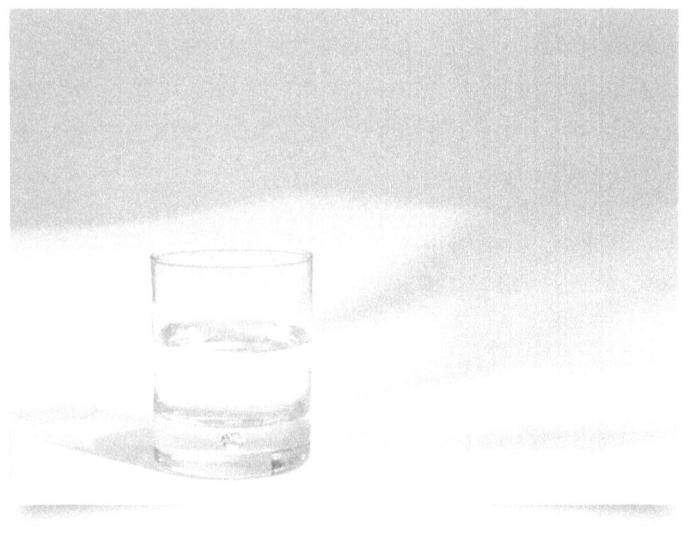

Photo by Manu Schwendener on Unsplash

Move

Often when I am delivering a session on neuroscience and wellbeing and get to the exercise part of the program, I ask the question: what's the best form of exercise? I usually get a range of responses and a laugh when I give the audience the answer: the one you will actually do.

I am not going to lecture you on the need for exercise. I am sure that the nagging voice inside your brain does enough of that. In the same way that you need to find which method of mindfulness works for you, you need to find the exercise that you can bring yourself to do regularly.

Remember, our brains evolved to move through our environment and experience new things. The key word is move, but how you move makes a big difference. The sedentary life that a lot of us find ourselves with, sitting or even standing in front of computer screens, is not conducive to either brain health or overall health.

Exercise does not just have physical benefits; it also has psychological and emotional benefits. If you can include a social component, even more rewards are reaped. And a little bit of exercise can go a long way, particularly if you are doing it regularly. Just a few extra or fewer steps each day can make a difference.

I discovered this thanks to COVID (the gift that keeps on giving . . . not). When I caught the bus or train into the Sydney CBD pre-COVID, I would walk from the train or bus station to the office and back again in the afternoon. Walking from my home-office (a slightly separate room in my house) to my home just wasn't the same. I was surprised at how much difference those extra steps had made.

Not only that, but the walk was also my transition time between work and home. On my walk into work, I was moving from home and 'off work' time and preparing for 'work' time. On the walk back, I did the opposite.

During lockdown, I had to develop different rituals to signal the end of the workday and the start of my 'home' time. These were no more complex than closing my laptop, turning off my home-office light and closing the door, but they were sufficient for me to feel that I could leave work at work.

If you are not prone to regular exercise and you want to start, that is going to be a habit change, so I recommend going back to the *Patterns and Habits* section and figuring out your Why, Will, and Way.

A word of caution; although you might think those devices that tell you the number of steps you are taking will help, they are a form of extrinsic motivation, and you will need to find your intrinsic motivation to have a lasting effect.

As with all patterns and habits, change takes time. What you tell yourself can also make a big difference. When I decided to write this book, instead of telling myself I was going to write, I told myself that I was a writer.

If you really want to start exercising, tell yourself 'I am a runner', or 'a walker', or 'a rower', or 'a boxer', or 'a pole dancer', or 'a kung fu initiate'. It changes your thinking and helps to motivate you by forming a connection to actually being that person. Words matter, especially self-talk - but more on this later.

Sleep

Having read and been deeply fascinated, and somewhat disturbed, by Mathew Walker's *Why We Sleep*, I could not leave sleep out of this book. It plays such an important role in our overall health, well-being, and longevity, and we spend a large part of our lives doing it, or trying to do it.

Sleep helps us to focus our AI. I read an article a while back that said that coming to work sleep deprived is as bad as, if not worse than, coming to work drunk, from a cognitive impairment perspective. Something to think about.

You may think that while you are sleeping, nothing is going on in your brain. In fact, there is a great deal going on in your brain that you are completely unaware of.

Your body has a system called the lymphatic system which drains impurities and allows white blood cells to travel around and fight invaders. It is the reason why doctors (and mothers) check under your jaw and sometimes your armpits, as the nodes of the lymphatic system become swollen when you are fighting an infection. They are also in your groin, but, fortunately for all involved, the neck area is more easily accessible.

It was thought for a long time that the brain had no way of clearing out damaged cells and toxins, as the lymphatic system does not run through there. Then, in 2015, the glymphatic system was discovered.

In your brain are other cells in addition to the neurons. One of these types of cells is called the glia cell. Glia is Latin for 'glue'. When we sleep, these glia cells shrink and allow glymphatic fluid to bathe the brain and wash away impurities. Think of it as a city at night. The glia cells open up pathways through the neurons to allow the street sweeper to pass and clean them up.

Sleep is a delicate balance of two things that have a much more pronounced effect on us than we may realise: hormones. Our old friend cortisol is involved, along with the hormone melatonin; you know, the one that makes it impossible to sleep when you have had a long plane flight and arrived at your destination and just want, but struggle to get, a good night's sleep before you explore? These two together are responsible for your circadian rhythm, which is supposed to put you to sleep when it is dark and wake you up when light. Core body temperature is also a key factor.

I'm going to go on a little tangent here, and possibly out on a limb, about teenagers, and say that not everything is their fault. They have a few things working against them. One is that their circadian rhythms are different to ours; they are off by about three hours, which makes them generally not at their best in the mornings.

This is why innovative schools around the world are looking into starting and ending the school day later for teenagers. I do wonder how the teachers, with their adult circadian rhythms, will feel about that. However, fortunately there is variation in the population between morning larks and night owls.

Adolescents have a few other factors going on in their brains that adults don't. The corpus collosum, a web that connects the left and right hemispheres of the brain, undergoes change in the teenage years. One of the functions of the corpus collosum is to connect consequences with actions. Of course, I have met quite a few adults who have a fully formed corpus collosum that is not, and probably never will be, fully functional, as they go on making poor choice after poor choice.

Teenagers also have some pruning going on while they sleep. Back to Hebb's law, the opposite also occurs, i.e., neurons that fire apart, wire apart. Those neuronal pathways that teenagers don't use frequently get pruned during sleep proving the adage 'use it or lose it'.

There are four stages of sleep which you cycle through as the night progresses:

Stage One - Rapid eye movement or REM sleep. Early in your sleep cycle, you tend to bounce up and down through the stages. The brain waves in REM sleep are quite fast, meaning the brain is still fairly active.

During this stage of sleep, we dream those fantastic dreams that seem to make no sense. REM sleep is vital for creativity, insight, innovation, and emotional regulation. It's REM sleep that can sometimes cause you to wake up with the solution to a problem you have been trying to solve.

Stage Two - This is the first of the non-REM sleep stages where brainwave activity starts to slow down. For the physics geeks, the frequency slows down and the amplitude increases.

Stages Three and Four - These stages combined are what is known as slow-wave sleep. Slow-wave sleep is critical for learning and memory consolidation. More on this in the section on learning. Generally, early in the night you bounce down into slow-wave sleep more than you do later in your night's sleep.

Gradually, as the night wears on and the hormones do their dance, you spend less and less time in slow-wave sleep and more time in stages one and two. Bottom line: all stages of sleep are vital to maintaining health and well-being.

OK, so what if you are the 3 a.m. waker? The problem is, our brain is not at its logical, reasoned best at 3 a.m. Both our physical and cognitive resources are low, and we have a tendency to exaggerate circumstances and catastrophise. This is really not helpful, certainly not conducive to going back to sleep, and can become a vicious cycle.

If the mindfulness technique you've found that works for you fails you on some of these occasions, there are a couple of other things you can try.

If you really can't get back to sleep because you are training your brain to be really good at worrying about that thing that happened a few days ago, have a note pad on hand. If you can, get up and write down the issue and possible solutions. This helps to get it out of your head.

If that doesn't work, you might try reading a book but they say it needs to be a real book, not an e-book. I recommend that, if you do read on your device, set it to a black background. I've found this allows me to read for a short period of time without getting out of bed, and I can focus on something other than that nagging problem. It provides a circuit breaker to the thinking. A side benefit is I don't disturb (and annoy) my husband by having to get out of bed or turn on an irritating light.

Another technique I have found that works is going to sound really weird, but bear with me. Have you ever 'looked' at the inside of your eyelids when your eyes are closed? When you focus on them, shapes start to appear and move around. I have found that doing this in the night can take my mind off the nagging thoughts circling my brain and the next thing I'm aware of is waking up in the morning. Remember, you need to find the techniques that work for you.

Finally, a word on napping; a little bit of sleep can go a long way. More and more workplaces are exploring putting in sleeping pods to assist in creativity and insight. When I worked for Microsoft in the early 90s and travelled to the mecca of Microsoft, Seattle, they had game rooms to facilitate down time, and it was not unheard of for programmers to be found curled up under tables taking a nanna nap.

There are levels of napping and benefits to each one:

- The power nap is a 10-20 minute nap where the goal is to stay in Stage Two. This helps to make you feel more alert, have more energy, and still process and consolidate some memories. Because you are only in Stage Two sleep, it is easier to wake up.

- The 60-minute nap is more about memory consolidation and has the same benefits as the power nap, but with the downside that you can awake feeling groggy.

- The 90-minute nap allows you to go through all stages of sleep. This nap has the benefits of the power and 60-minute nap, improving skill and procedural memory, problem solving, and creativity. And, you awake feeling refreshed.

So, nanna had it right after all.

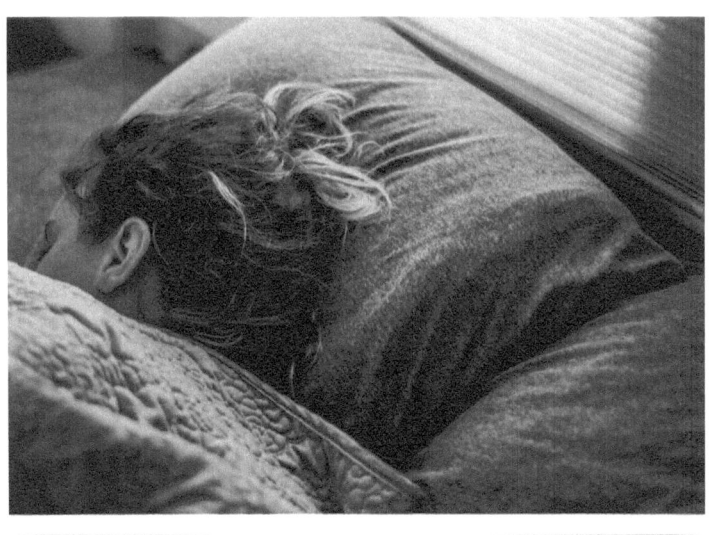

Photo by Gregory Pappas on Unsplash

Part 3: Where to from here?

Put your own oxygen mask on first

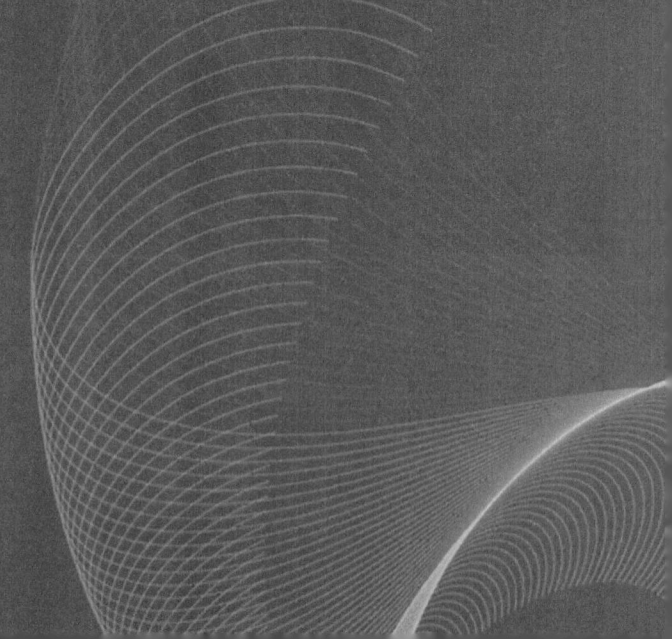

So, you've made it this far on the journey and hopefully learned some things, relearned some things you had forgotten, or maybe determined to unlearn some things that you have held onto past their use-by date.

Before we get into the next part, and, yes, slightly randomly, I want to have a word about inflammation. Chronic inflammation affects brain structure. Not only that, but inflammation in general can be stealthy and damaging to the body as a whole.

When I was teaching biology, I read an article regarding the immune system of children who grow up on farms and have more faecal material in their environment in general; even in their bedding. These children tended to have much more robust and less over-reactive immune systems than children who grew up in more sterile conditions.

More recently, I saw an article that referred to research by Barbara Fredrickson from the University of North Carolina at Chapel Hill and Steve Cole from UCLA on levels of happiness and meaningful lives, as self-reported by 80 research subjects.

If you have a history of loneliness, social isolation, and other adversity, your immune system response is to prepare you for bacterial infections that your ancestors may have historically gotten as a consequence of wounding in battles and hunts. However, the immune system in those people who haven't had adversity in their lives, and have good, healthy social relationships, is better prepared for viral infections due to the increased social interactions. Their research found that people who reported they were happy but had no meaning in their life had immune systems that were prepared for bacterial infections.

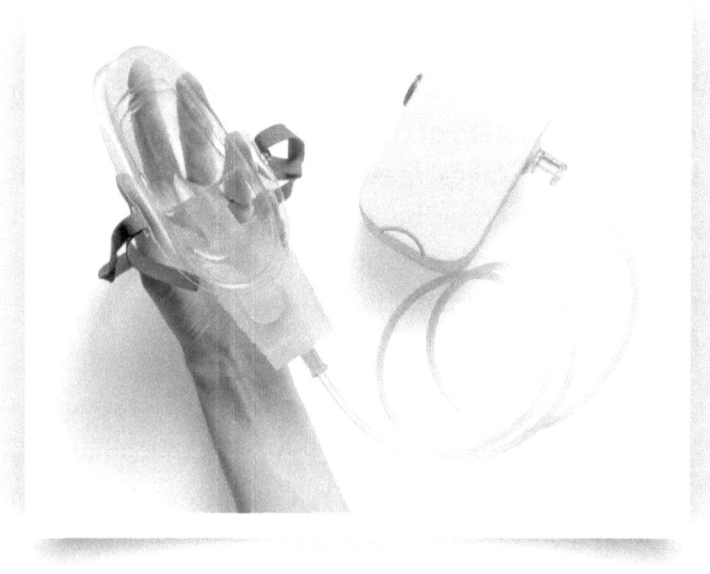

Photo by Mockup Graphics on Unsplash

Along the lines of the 'put your own oxygen mask on first' principle, you can't be a good partner, parent, relative, or friend if you are not in the right headspace or dealing with yourself first.

Part 3 is about how to develop and flex some of the skills that will help you and your brain navigate the next part of your journey, whatever that may be and wherever that may lead you.

Resilience

Like the rest of the world, I have found the past few years with COVID to be somewhat challenging. Yes, we may all be in the same boat, but everyone's context and experience is different, and so each of us has responded in different ways.

We each entered the situation with different amounts of baggage, coping thresholds, and life experience. We all have different levels of resilience based on that baggage, our patterns and habits, and past experiences.

Resilience, like patterns and habits, is partly genetically pre-determined, and, after that, is based on your personality and temperament. However, like empathy, resilience can be learned, and you can build your resilience muscle through conscious focus and attentional intelligence.

One of the issues we have had with the pandemic is not knowing what will happen next. This degree of uncertainty causes our predicting brain to be stressed. A stressed brain is flooded with cortisol, and we find it hard to make decisions, particularly in the spur of the moment.

Because of their genetics, personality, and temperament, some people will deal with this stress better than others, but often the longer the uncertainty goes on, the more stressed we tend to become.

The interesting thing about stress is that it is our perception of it that makes the difference. There is a bell curve of perceived stress, and different people will be at different points based on their past experiences, personality, and temperament.

We all know the person who seems to go off at the smallest thing. They are what we used to call in IBM at the 'bleeding edge' (as opposed to leading edge) of the bell curve. Then there are others who seem to have five of the top most stressful things happening at once and sail on through with impressive equanimity. The rest of us tend to fall somewhere in the middle.

I heard a great concept a while ago that was about 'certainty buckets'. Basically, if you have two buckets, one labelled 'certainty' and one labelled 'uncertainty', it is about balance. If your certainty bucket is reasonably full, you can deal with a level of uncertainty. If, however, your certainty bucket is depleted, the smallest amount of uncertainty can seem overwhelming.

It doesn't have to be large-scale things that can fill your certainty bucket. It could be as simple as knowing what you are going to wear into the office the next day (there's the argument for uniforms) or what you will have for lunch. The more you fill your certainty bucket, the better able you are to deal with the uncertainty that gets thrown at you.

Many moons ago, I read a book that changed the way I approached work and life: Stephen R. Covey's *The 7 Habits of Highly Effective People*. I still use a 7 Habits organiser today. Covey talked about the circle of control, the circle of influence, and the circle of concern:

The inner circle; the circle of control - things that are within my control to change.

The middle circle; the circle of influence - things I cannot directly control but may be able to influence the outcomes of based on my relationships or actions.

The outer circle; here's where I deviate a bit from Covey's circle of concern. I call this the circle of 'stop waking at three in the morning and worrying about it' - things I cannot control or influence and have to leave to external factors to deal with.

When you realise this, you can respond to the things that are in your control and influence and leave the rest to sort themselves out one way or another. This gives you a level of certainty, and even freedom, because you know what issues you can manage directly and which ones you have to let go of. You have choices.

A couple of years ago, I had the good fortune to hear Christine Nixon (the former Chief Commissioner of Victoria Police) speak. Christine had an interesting career that started as a policewoman in Sydney's notorious Kings Cross. She is a highly resilient woman who tells some gritty stories of her time as one of the few women in the police force in the 70s.

One of the stories she told was about the 1.6m wall that would-be police recruits had to scale as part of their training. When, as the Chief Police Commissioner, it became clear to her that women were not making it through the academy because they couldn't scale the wall, she instructed them to remove the wall. She argued that, in a pursuit, not one police man or woman she knew had to scale a 1.6m wall and that it was stopping otherwise solid recruits from making it onto the police force.

I have a concept I call parkour (you know, that crazy sport of running and jumping and climbing over obstacles) leadership. This is the idea that, as a leader, you need to be able to go over, under, around, or through obstacles. You can also remove barriers to what you need to achieve, as Christine did with the wall. Too often we look to add something to solve problems, as opposed to a reductionist view that asks: what can we remove to solve this? Think of the balance bike. This brilliant solution, rather than adding on training wheels, involves making the bike small enough to allow the child to place their feet on the ground. I watched my grandson, at the ripe old age of three, go barrelling down our driveway on the balance bike like a pro after a matter of days.

Resilience is not only how you handle adversity, but also how quickly you recover from it. Another quintessential book I read in the early 90s was *Learned Optimism* by Martin Seligman. Seligman talks about the three Ps: permanence, pervasiveness, and personalisation. People who see adversity as lasting forever, affecting everything in their lives, and being all about them are more pessimistic and not as resilient.

The point of his book is in the title. Like empathy and resilience, optimism can be learned. The corollary of learned optimism is, as Seligman put it, learned helplessness. It, too, is a skill that can be learned and become a debilitating pattern or habit that makes us less resilient. Helplessness or optimism is a choice we can make as to what we respond with in any given situation.

In January 2021, before I came up with my SOLAR © framework, I had decided that the year was going to be my year of decluttering and reframing, or reappraisal, as it is also called. During COVID, I worked on a cross-stitch of the kings and queens of England I had bought 20 years before and never got around to; it was ridiculously small stitching and so I had put it off, very successfully. It became my COVID cross-stitch challenge, and I managed to finally complete it late in 2020.

On a sunny day in January 2021, right before returning to work, I was driving to take it to a framer to get it mounted to give to my gorgeous grandson who is partially (and serendipitously) named after one of the kings. On the way there, I was listening to the radio and not really concentrating on my driving (thank goodness for my patterns and habits).

In Australia, we have these rather large hairy spiders called huntsman spiders. Whilst largely harmless, they are quite freaky, particularly if you are not a huge fan of spiders (Give me a red-belly black snake any day!). I'm driving along and one runs down my windscreen.

My thoughts ran like this (the voice in your head reading this needs to be at very high volume):

'Oh expletive, oh expletive, oh expletive!'

'Is it on the inside?????'

'Of course it's not on the inside!!!'

'Oh no, it's gone under the bonnet!'

'It's going to come through the aircon vents.'

'Of course it can't do that . . . can it?'

'I want to get out of the car RIGHT NOW!!!'

'You can't do that, you're travelling at 60kms an hour, not to mention driving.'

'But I really, really want to get out.'

'Well you can't, so suck it up. You think you're so clever, Ms Neuroscience nerd, reframe this one.'

'Ok . . . what would the spider be thinking right now?'

'Oh expletive, oh expletive, oh expletive! I'm on a car going 60 kms an hour!!!'

At that point I laughed. The thing is, it made me relax enough to stay in the car, drive in a seemingly responsible way, get to my destination and then leap out of the car like a mad woman rather than jumping out of it at 60kms an hour.

Reframing is a powerful neuroscience technique you can use in the moment to be more resilient.

Having a growth mindset is also important for resilience. Given voice by Carol Dweck in her book Mindset, it is, at its essence, the idea that you can develop and hone talents with learning. It's summed up by the phrase 'it's not that I can't do something, it's that I can't do it YET'.

Cognitive flexibility is something that can be learned and helps to make you more resilient. This is the ability to adapt to circumstances and come up with creative solutions. It has more to do with what is called fluid intelligence, and is mostly independent from IQ.

It is important to build and flex your resilience muscle regularly. Challenge yourself and try something different, or something you have been putting off doing for fear of failure. Accept that there may be setbacks that you can learn from and try again. Having something to look forward to, such as a specific event, and visualising that event also helps to build the resilience muscle. Resilient people, like people with purpose, tend to be healthier, happier, and live longer.

Purpose

I deliberated long and hard about including this part in the book. Purpose, or meaning, has been written about and expounded on since the days of Seneca, and probably before. I finally decided that I would include a bit on it, and do so by telling my purpose story. You may have figured out by now that I am a bit of a storyteller.

When I first started running leadership development programs, I attended a session being delivered by one of my colleagues. She is someone who earned her master's degree at the Harvard Kennedy School of Government and for whom I have enormous regard. While she was there, she spent a year as the lead teaching assistant with the guru of adaptive leadership, Professor Ronald Heifetz.

In the session I attended, my colleague (and now friend) was unpacking one of the concepts of adaptive leadership around leadership versus authority. As part of it, she ran an activity where we had to choose a fictional or non-fictional character that we admired. We then wrote down three reasons why we admired them. The character I chose was Ellen Ripley from the Alien movie series. My husband was a huge fan and insisted that I watch every one of them, which I did through the filter of my fingers.

> I am not a huge fan of gory movies. Strange, I hear you say, given I have a degree in biology and have no doubt done many dissections. I am also that person who has the uncanny ability to come across accidents as they are happening or shortly thereafter.
>
> Consequently, I have maintained my first aid certificate over the years because I figured, if I had to be that person, I might as well know what to do to help. Real life gore I can deal with; Hollywood, not so much. Weird, huh?

I chose Ripley for these three reasons:

1. She stepped up.

2. She kicked butt.

3. She did it even when she was scared.

My colleague then went on to explain the Jungian concept of the Golden Shadow. This is the idea that what we admire most in others lies deep within ourselves. When I told her who I had chosen and why, she said, 'Yep, that's you, Jen. That's what you do'.

Move forward a few years and we were running sessions helping school leaders to identify their purpose. There is a great Harvard Business Review article from Nick Craig and Scott Snook titled *From Purpose to Impact*, which I highly recommend. As a team, we decided that we needed to practice what we preach, and went through the activities in the article to try to draw out our individual purpose.

This purpose is not just from a work perspective, but permeates all that we do and drives why we get out of bed in the morning. In conversations with my colleague and friend, I realised I had already landed on my purpose with Ripley. When I was stepping up and handling situations, even when I really didn't want to, I found I was energised and firing on all six cylinders.

So, if I am uncertain about what to do next, I ask myself: 'What would Ripley do?' Of course, I generally don't have to deal with aliens (although there are times when it feels like it), but it reminds me to step up and deal with whatever 'it' is, nonetheless.

People with purpose are less stressed and more resilient. They have lower levels of cortisol, cholesterol, and inflammation. Having purpose gives them a reason for doing things and comes with a nice hit of the feelgood hormone, dopamine.

So, I encourage you to find, or perhaps re-find, your purpose, to reenergise and refocus if you have lost direction.

The final part...

'A jack of all trades is a master of none, but oftentimes better than a master of one.'

William Shakespeare

Love, laugh, and live

Recently I was reflecting on a time when I was the parent of a young child (a long time ago, as my 'baby' is now mid-twenties), a step-mum to three gorgeous kids, a business owner, CFO, and consultant in that same business. I felt like my brain was only firing on three cylinders instead of the six it used to, and I was so busy being a mum, wife, step-mum, company director, consultant, etc., that I couldn't complete a full sentence. The last person to cross my mind was me.

That's not to say that being a mum and a step-mum wasn't both a gift and a joy. It did mean, though, that I was so busy thinking of everyone else, I forgot that in order to be the best mum, wife, businesswoman, and so on and so forth, I needed to carve out the time to put me first sometimes. That's not selfish, that's smart, and also good parenting. Remember the oxygen mask?

Children learn a lot by watching. Whether we are conscious of it or not, we model resilience, perseverance, and work ethic, amongst other things, and they watch and learn. Their patterns and habits can come about because of what they see growing up. Children as young as 15 months can observe adults working towards a particular goal and mimic the behaviour. It's a heck of a responsibility for adults, and one we need to be conscious of.

When it comes to love, I am not going to enter the realms of romance novelists (although I did dabble at one stage) or great love stories (not even thinking about going there). I will, however, talk a little about self-love and that annoying little voice we all have in our heads: self-talk.

Because the brain is so focussed on survival, in the absence of information it will fill in the gaps with a negative storyline. In addition to this, we (mostly) all suffer, at times, from imposter syndrome. Your self-talk is very important to your motivation and how you show up in different situations.

Amy Cuddy, the American Social Psychologist, has a saying: 'Fake it till you become it.' The words that you use, even to yourself, matter. There is a difference, though, between self-talk designed to move you to a better place and self-talk that is essentially kidding yourself. Full confession time: there have been times in my life when I have tried to fool myself and tell myself a story that I would like to believe was true. I have learned that it's wise not to try to fool yourself; sooner or later you'll figure out what you are trying to do!

Try keeping a journal with what you say to others and what you say to yourself. Someone I know who did this was shocked at how positive he was to others and how negative he was to himself.

There is a spectrum of how people see the future. Some take the view that what they do today will influence the future, while others have the view that nothing they do will change what will happen to them. Self-talk has a lot to do with where you sit on that spectrum, and there are times when you need to take that annoying voice firmly in hand and tell it to just be quiet.

Sometimes laughter, even if, or perhaps especially if, you are the butt (no pun intended) of it, can indeed be the best medicine. Although, there will be times in life where you can't see the humour in anything. It also depends on your outlook; are you a glass-half-full or glass-half-empty type of person? I once described someone as not only being a glass-half-empty type, but letting someone else drink what was left. That's a pretty sad and debilitating view of life.

Here's the thing; being miserable takes energy, particularly if you are trying to sustain it for any length of time. I have seen several people in my life who have had good and justifiable cause to be miserable, and yet chose to use that energy to turn their lives around.

My longest-term (I refuse to say 'oldest') and closest friend became so in a pivotal moment (you have no idea how much I looked for an alternate word here as I learned to hate the word 'pivot' in 2020 through gross overuse and misuse, but this is actually the correct word for the moment).

I had known her for many years, as we had been to the same schools, and were friendly but not especially close. We were sitting at the train station in our penultimate year of school, when hormones are raging and image is all. Whatever was said, her response was to push me, which resulted in me sliding off the bench and landing, butt first, in a small, round garbage bin. Picture ultimate humiliation and total teenage embarrassment. I had a choice: rant and rail, or laugh. I chose to laugh. In that moment, a lifetime friendship was forged. One that has seen us through tragic lows and heart-warming highs.

Self-directed neuroplasticity is the idea that you can direct where your attention and focus are aimed. Think of the algorithms underpinning Facebook and Google, where every time you do a search they pick up what you've been looking at and give you suggestions and advertising based on your searches and likes.

In the same way, if you focus your attention on certain things, your brain gets the message that it must be important, and so your attention is drawn to that. For example, have you ever been thinking of buying a particular type of car and then, all of a sudden, you seem to see them everywhere? It's not that there are more of those cars on the road, it's that you are noticing them because you have focussed your attention on them. You can choose where you focus your attention, for good or ill, which is attentional intelligence.

There is ongoing research around a collection of brain regions known as the default mode network, or DMN. These regions are active when we are not engaged in specific thinking or physical activities; the research has shown that we are in DMN around 47% of the time.

There are hypotheses as to the DMN's role in the social brain, as well as in relation to diseases such as Alzheimer's. In order to actively engage your attentional intelligence, you need to consciously disengage your default mode network.

Attentional intelligence is about harnessing the superpower that is your brain, and its plasticity, to determine not only the pathway that you are on in life, but where that pathway goes and how to move the path around, over, under, or through the obstacles that you encounter on the journey. I call this parkour leadership. You can't change the past, and you can't predict the future (although the brain is constantly trying to); you can only be in the present.

There's a great concept that has been around for a long time: eudaimonia. Used back in the time of Aristotle (although, despite what some of my students thought, I wasn't around to verify that), central to this concept is the idea of striving based on your own unique potential and flourishing in the process.

Shakespeare's usually truncated quote of 'A jack of all trades is a master of none' actually ends with 'but oftentimes better than a master of one.' It was intended as a compliment.

So, try your hand at many things.

Get outside and move through your environment.

Dance a little, sing a little, laugh a little.

Always keep learning.

Remember to breathe. And live a lot.

Appendices

Appendix A: SOLAR ©

Appendix B: BLAISE ©

Appendix C: All the brilliant books I recommend

Appendix A: SOLAR © A framework for leading in uncertain times

I live in Sydney and in this not-quite-post-pandemic world I drive into the city instead of using the bus. In February 2021, as I was driving in to deliver our first leadership program of the year, I came across the Harbour Bridge and was sitting at the traffic lights at the start of York Street. I had been bouncing ideas around in my head based on the latest lectures I had been listening to. I was thinking about our patterns and habits and different strategies and techniques; how they would interplay with each other and how you could deploy them in the heat of the moment.

I had already decided that 2021, off the back of 2020, was going to be my year of reframing, which is a neuroscience technique for viewing a situation from a more objective perspective. As I sat at the lights, I had an 'aha' moment. These moments arise when you have been focussed on a problem or a conundrum but are not directly focussing on it at that time. Have you ever had a solution to a problem come to you when you first wake up? Or when you are out walking, or in the shower? That's an aha moment.

From my aha moment, a single neuroscience framework coalesced: SOLAR ©. So here it is.

We live in a **VUCA (Volatile, Uncertain, Complex, Ambiguous)** world. Intellectually, I knew that, and then 2020 happened. Now I understand on a visceral level what it really means.

That year provided a burning platform for change on a daily (and sometimes hourly) basis. Any change can be seen by the brain as a threat, so in 2020, with the levels of uncertainty we all experienced, there were times when we may have felt overwhelmed, particularly as the situation unfolded.

In the absence of information, as a survival mechanism, most of us will fill in the blanks with a negative story. While this may have helped us avoid the sabre-tooth in the bushes in the past, generally this is not something we need to worry about anymore. However, the context we find ourselves in, the facial expressions, body language, and words that people use, can be seen by the brain as a threat.

In uncertain times, we are more anxious, don't sleep as well, and have a tendency to ruminate or wallow in the negative. This can lead to a downward spiral that means we focus on the problem, not potential solutions, and are in our limbic system. When we are in our limbic system, we are experiencing emotions that can heighten our anxiety and keep us in the downward spiral.

SOLAR © is a framework based on neuroscience techniques that can help you stop the downward spiral, move from the limbic to the prefrontal cortex, and focus on a different way of looking at the situation. This allows you to better navigate a way forward in uncertain times.

S - Stop. Literally, stop the thinking. If you go over and over a situation, you are simply strengthening your neural pathways to be extremely good at worrying. You are also reliving the moment, complete with the emotions you experienced at the time. Say it out loud if you can (without scaring small children).

O - Observe. What are the emotions you are experiencing? Pull them into the light and examine them. Sit with them for a minute until you recognise them.

L - Label. When you recognise the emotions you're feeling, give them a name. Naming and claiming them is a well-researched technique for viewing your emotions from a more objective perspective, thus moving you from your limbic to your PFC. It's like taking a mental step back from them.

A - Ask. Ask yourself some questions: Do I have all the information? What information might I be missing? Have I just had a bad day/week/month (or in the case of 2020, year)? Am I viewing this situation from a negative standpoint because of past interactions?

R - Reframe. This is another powerful neuroscience technique. Sometimes called reappraisal, it is about taking a different perspective on a situation. How can you view the situation differently? How can you learn from it so you show up differently next time? If someone else was looking at the situation, what would they see? This deploys what is called the 'high road' in the brain, which gives you the ability to see things from a more objective perspective and make more strategic decisions.

So go ahead, give it a go. You may not work through every step each time, but it is a framework that you can use in most circumstances to take control of your thoughts and literally change your brain.

Appendix B: BLAISE © The neuroscience of learning

BLAISE © is an acronym that you can use to remember how to design and deliver professional learning with the brain in mind.

Brain - Learning involves your working memory (in your PFC), short-term memory (hippocampus) and your long-term memory (hippocampus and cortex). I suggest you re-read A quick tour of the Brain in Part 1 if you need to refresh yourself on the function, affiliations, and location of these parts of the brain.

There are two types of intelligence: fluid intelligence and crystallized intelligence. Fluid intelligence is the ability to reason and synthesise, and is processed via your working memory. Crystallized intelligence is accumulated as you go through life and comprises the facts, figures, and knowledge that you gain and store in long-term memory.

Learning - We learn by taking input from our senses, processing via our working memory, making connections with past experiences and knowledge, and then processing the new information we want to hold onto into long-term memory via the hippocampus.

The brain is constantly taking input, detecting patterns, making connections and meaning, and predicting what will happen next based on that. The brain is also constantly alert for new and novel experiences.

When a prediction is not fulfilled, we come out of our long-term memory and into our working memory again. A lot of this is occurring at the sub-conscious level, and so a level of meta-cognition is required to challenge our predictions.

For us to be in the learning zone, we need to have the following conditions:

- Between threat and reward - The brain learns best when you are slightly stressed but not feeling threatened. Eustress (a positive form of stress) enhances attention, focus and memory retention.

- Between fear and boredom - Emotions are part of learning; a slightly positive state is better than a negative state although both are conducive to learning. Too much emotional arousal is not good for memory retention, creativity, or collaboration.

- When we are not overly anxious, we are able to pay attention. By reducing anxiety in a learning situation, you can gain people's attention and help them focus.

Attentional Intelligence - Where you focus your working memory is where you will learn. In a learning situation, multitasking impairs both your learning and the learning of those within eyesight of your multitasking.

Because emotions focus your attention and assist in processing what you learn into long-term memory, as well as in the importance of our social brain, storytelling can be a very effective way to help people learn. Through hearing others' stories, they can recall their own experiences and see themselves in these stories, engaging their emotions. This reflection helps them to make meaning of the new learning.

Spacing - Remember Goldilocks? Your PFC gets tired at around the 20-minute mark, which means your working memory doesn't work so well after that without a break. Chunking allows people to engage their working memory and then have time to process what they have learned.

Spacing can also extend over several days; in fact, learning is better when there is time for them to think about what they have learned, discuss it with others, and make connections with what they have learned. The best way to learn something is to teach it to others.

Sleep is the other factor that is part of spacing and enhances learning significantly. Have a look at the *Sleep* section in Part 2, concerning the importance of sleep in processing what we learn into long-term memory.

Emergence - If you've ever had a moment when you are immersed in something but thinking about it peripherally, perhaps even dreaming about it, and then come up with a completely new idea, that's emergence. My SOLAR © framework, and to a lesser extent BLAISE ©, came from there. It's those aha moments or moments of insight when a completely new idea emerges that is different from, but often a synthesis of, what you have learned. The concept of emergence is beautifully explained and illustrated in Jared Cooney Horvath's book *Stop Talking, Start Influencing*.

We learn, reflect on what we have learned, and make connections with past experiences and knowledge. Designing learning experiences with an understanding of the brain, how it learns, how it focusses attention, how space is required for the connections to be made leads to insights from which new things emerge.

As educators, it is our responsibility to develop experiences that enhance learning and foster a love of learning. If we keep learning as we go through life, not only does it energise us, strengthen the brain, and improve overall health and wellbeing, but it can help us to live longer.

When I was growing up, I often heard George Bernard Shaw's line 'Those who can, do; those who can't, teach'. I always thought it maligned teachers. When I became a teacher myself, I had a new understanding of its meaning. Just because you are good at something, doesn't mean you can teach it. It takes a special type of person to be able to understand something well enough to teach it to others. My hat goes off to all of you. Keep up the good fight because you do make a difference; you just may not know it until a long time later.

I was recently at a medical facility having one of the many tests that aging inflicts upon us (mind you, the alternative is worse!) and, as it was still in the times of COVID, was diligently wearing my mask. At the end, when I went to the counter with my little slip of paper that dictated whether or not our government would cover my expenses or my private enterprise would, the young woman behind the counter asked me if

I had taught at a particular school previously. I told her I had, and she informed me that I had been her biology teacher. I was delighted and congratulated her on recognising me with my mask on, to which she replied, 'Well, your name is up on the screen'. OK, duh.

Anyway, she said that biology had been her favourite subject and went on to let me know that she was just finishing up her medical degree. It's those moments that remind us why we went into education in the first place.

Appendix C: All the brilliant books I recommend

Atomic Habits by James Clear

Breath by James Nestor

Indistractable by Nir Eyal

Learned Optimism by Martin Seligman

Mindset by Carol Dweck

Stop Talking, Start Influencing by Jared Cooney Horvath

The Brain That Changes Itself by Norman Doidge

The 7 Habits of Highly Effective People by Stephen R. Covey

Thinking, Fast and Slow by Daniel Kahneman

Why We Sleep by Mathew Walker

Your Brain at Work by David Rock

www.ingramcontent.com/pod-product-compliance
Lightning Source LLC
Chambersburg PA
CBHW030306100526
44590CB00012B/545